The Essential Diet:
Eating for Mental Health

Dr. Christina Bjorndal, ND

For additional information or wholesale orders, please email:
admin@naturalterrain.com and put THE ESSENTIAL DIET in the subject line
or contact the Natural Terrain Naturopathic Clinic
#200 - 6650 177th St NW, Edmonton, AB T5T 4J5

Library and Archive Canada Cataloguing in Publication

Bjorndal, Christina, 1967-
The Essential Diet: Eating for Mental Health / Christina Bjorndal

ISBN: 978-1-77084-948-8

1. Cookery (Natural foods) 2. Mental Health
Cover and design by Rana Keen-Zandbeek
Edited by Alexis Rebeyka and Lachlan Crawford
Photography by Shutterstock and Pexels
Back cover photography by Rana Keen-Zandbeek

Printed and bound in Canada by First Choice Books

Contents

Acknowledgments

This book is the combination of many years of study, clinical experience, inspiration, perseverance and trial and error. I owe gratitude to many people who have influenced my career and naturopathic philosophy in guiding patients to regain their mental health.

Thank you to my husband, Dr. Michael Mason-Wood, who is the true creative force behind this book. He is the imaginative cook and master gardener in our family. I know the food you grow, the recipes you create and the meals you make are infused with your love for us. Your unconditional love and support is not lost on me. Thank you for always encouraging me to reach new heights, to step into the places that scare me and to be that gentle hand on my back supporting me. I love you.

A special thank you to my parents. Mom, for everything...really. You are an amazing cook and I only wish I had been open to learning our family recipes from you while growing up versus being more interested in sports and studying! Every meal you made for me nourished my mind, body and spirit. Dad, for teaching me about work ethic and business. You have always been a steady, calm, gentle and strong force in my life. I would not be the person I am today if I hadn't had you both as parents. I love you.

Preface

When I first went to see a Naturopathic Doctor in 1996, I had to cut out wheat, dairy, sugar, chocolate, eggs and tomatoes from my diet. My response was "What's left to eat?!" At that time, I knew very little about diet, nutrition or healthy eating. I certainly didn't know what quinoa was, where to find it, how to cook it or even how to spell or pronounce it. In fact, I didn't even know that there were other grains to eat except wheat and rice. Over the past 20 years, I have slowly made changes to my diet. I feel the best I have ever felt as I enter my fifties. And you can too! The key is awareness. Awareness of how food makes you feel. In time, you will make healthier choices because you simply feel better doing so.

When it comes to eating, I am not an extremist. I have had an eating disorder and my philosophy with food is that ultimately what you eat and how you treat your body is a reflection of how you feel about yourself. Follow the 80-90/20-10 rule ~ 80-90% of the time you eat according to the healthy plan and 10-20% of the time you might not. The goal is not perfection. Enjoyment is! I want you to enjoy what you eat. Don't eat guilt, shame and blame along with that organic dark chocolate bar. It is my goal to help you feel better using food. Food is the fuel that provides the building blocks for you to make neurotransmitters - such as the "feel good" neurotransmitter serotonin - which is needed to prevent depression and anxiety. I often say to patients "If you don't put the right gas in the car, the car is not going to run properly".

Preparation, and taking the time to prepare, is key. Eating healthfully requires prioritization and organization. Take the time to go grocery shopping so that your fridge and pantry are stocked with the items you need (see grocery shopping lists pages 9 - 12). I often double the recipe so I have leftovers and don't have to cook every night. Use this guide in a way that works best for you!

You will have more energy, sleep better, have a clearer mind, and improved digestion if you follow the Essential Diet. This is your guide to eating for mental well-being. Start where you can. Do what you can. You've got this! Enjoy!

Dr. Chris

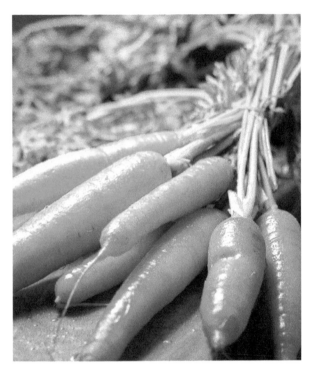
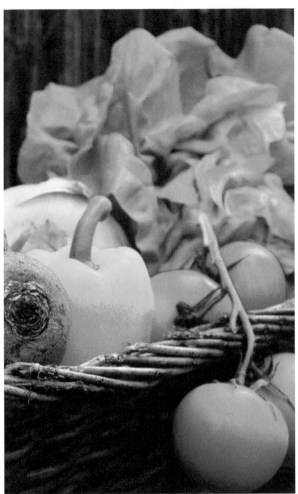
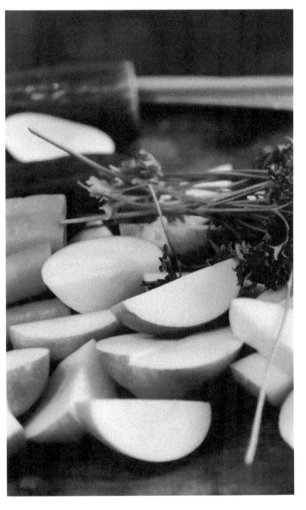
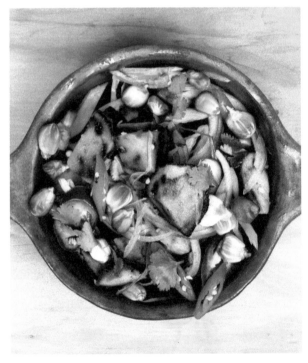

There is a growing body of scientific evidence that voices support for the age-old idea that what we eat affects both our bodies and our minds. Not only can a supportive diet maintain the physical body, it is also important when it comes to our mental health. In fact, our diet patterns can hugely impact our minds, influencing our daily moods and how we interact with the world. The fact that food is so emotionally potent is empowering; each of us has the ability to modify our diet to benefit our bodies and minds. When eating for physical and mental health, there are some guidelines to help you make choices and form good habits for a healthy mind and body.

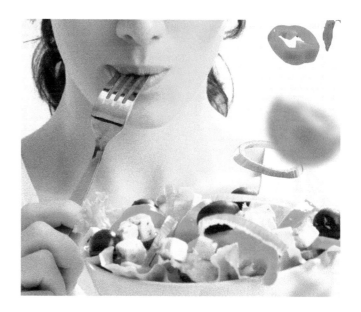

One of the most important ways our diet impacts our moods is through our blood sugar levels. High spikes in these levels immediately after a sugary or high-carbohydrate meal may feel briefly energizing, but is inevitably followed by a drop in blood sugar levels. This causes our energy to plummet, impacting our mood and making us irritable. It can also contribute to headaches, fatigue and dizziness. Regularly having high-sugar foods can condition us to want more and create a sugar addiction. This cycle makes us reach for sugar to make us feel better without considering the blood sugar crash that will follow. Keeping an eye on sugar and carbohydrates is a good way to regulate your mood throughout the day.

On food labels, sugar is quoted in grams. But what does this really mean? When reading labels, it is important to know that 4 grams of sugar equals 1 teaspoon. For example, if the yogurt you are eating is artificially sweetened, it may contain 24 grams of sugar in a ½ cup serving. This is the equivalent of 6 tsp of sugar, which is a lot! In this case, it is better to buy plain yogurt and mix in ½ a cup of fresh fruit.

Pay attention to your current daily intake of added sugar (i.e. found in packaged products with refined sugar) and try not to exceed 24 grams (6 teaspoons) for women and 36 grams (9 teaspoons) for men. See page 4 for tips on how to eliminate sugar.

Another way to use food as a tool for mental health is to eat mindfully. Huge benefits are possible when one pays special attention to the act of eating: from a greater enjoyment of the food to enhanced digestion and better absorption of nutrients. Several resources are available to help you develop a habit of eating mindfully such as Thich Nhat Hanh's book *Savor*. Start by doing nothing else while you eat. Clean your desk or table, put away your phone, move away from your computer and sit quietly with your meal. Pay attention with all your senses: How does the food smell? How does it look? How does it sound as your utensil clinks on the plate? How does it feel in your mouth and as you swallow? And of course, how does it taste? Breathe deeply, chew slowly, 30-50 times per bite and finish swallowing a mouthful before you reach for another bite. Start this practice with one meal a day and observe how it affects your enjoyment of eating and your digestion afterwards. If sharing your meal with someone, develop a practice of spending the first few minutes eating mindfully together then be social for the rest of the meal. You'll be surprised how this habit can even help you to be mindful in other areas of your life.

For mental well-being and weight management, there are many theories about what to eat and what not to eat. It is my intention to make this clear and easy for you. Simply put, you need to ensure that your diet incorporates all the essential macromolecules or nutritional building blocks that your body requires to make the neurotransmitters and hormones that are responsible for a balanced mood. These include:

• Essential amino acids involved in neurotransmitter formation: tryptophan for serotonin and phenylalanine for dopamine
• Essential fats involved in both neurotransmitter and hormone formation: omega 3 and omega 6
• Nutrients involved in neurotransmitter formation: vitamin B3, vitamin B6, magnesium, vitamin C, vitamin D and zinc

Food has a significant influence on the brain's behaviour. A poor diet, especially one high in junk food, is a common cause of mental dis-ease. The levels of neurotransmitters are controlled by what we eat. One very important neurotransmitter is serotonin as it plays a role in mood, sleep and appetite. Low levels of serotonin may result from diets too high in simple sugars/carbohydrates (e.g., white sugar, white flour, sweets, processed foods) and lead to depression, anxiety, binge eating and sleep disturbances. Diets high in complex carbohydrates (e.g., vegetables, whole grains, peas, and beans), on the other hand, help to increase serotonin and elevate mood.

Serotonin is derived from the essential amino acid tryptophan. By increasing tryptophan-containing foods, we can increase the amount of serotonin made in the brain. I struggled with my mental health for over fifteen years and in that time, not one doctor ever asked me what I was eating. When I was studying Naturopathic medicine, we had to analyze our diets for a nutrition assignment. I was shocked to discover that the only essential amino acid that I was deficient in was tryptophan. This was one of the reasons my mental health improved when I changed my diet and supplemented with vitamins and minerals because now the tryptophan pathway in my body was being supported.

If your diet currently consists of the following:
Breakfast: Tim Horton's Hot Breakfast Sandwich and a large double double
Lunch: Wendy's Dave Single Burger, large fries and pop
Dinner: Spaghetti and meatballs

then you may find the Essential Diet, as well as the foods to avoid suggestions, overwhelming. After my first visit to a Naturopathic Doctor it was prescribed that I cut out: wheat, dairy, sugar, chocolate, tomatoes and eggs. I found myself saying "what's left to eat"? This was also in the mid-90s long before there was any information about the negative effects of wheat and gluten-free products were practically non-existent in mainstream grocery stores. I also didn't know what quinoa was, and I certainly couldn't pronounce it or spell it.

At that time, my diet consisted of a piece of fruit for breakfast; I usually ate out for lunch – sometimes fast food, Subway or a healthier meal if I was taken out for lunch; and dinner was either a can of soup or a potato cooked in the microwave with grated cheddar cheese and salsa on top. I lived in my apartment for eight years and rarely used my oven. When I got married, I had never cooked a turkey or a roast. Simply put, I didn't know how to cook as I was too busy climbing the corporate ladder to care.

So I hear you. I get it. I've been there. If you are new to the concept of healthy eating then my suggestion is to incorporate one meal or snack per day from the Essential Diet. Cooking is easy. You've got this. It doesn't have to be complicated. Focus on the positive suggestions around food, such as increasing foods with tryptophan or foods high in essential fatty acids. In time, these will push out the "bad" food choices. I keep my meals simple: a protein (chicken, turkey or wild fish), a complex carbohydrate (brown rice or quinoa) and lots of vegetables. The key is to start where it feels possible for you. Use the general eating guidelines for balanced mental health as a place to start.

Get curious.
Try new things.
Experiment.
Make cooking fun!

General eating guidelines for balanced mental health:

1. Eat a variety of local fresh, unprocessed and unpackaged foods.

2. Strictly limit sugars and sugary foods. These simple carbohydrates or sugars initially increase energy, but it is quickly followed by fatigue and depression. Sugar also depletes the body of B vitamins and magnesium which are crucial to the production of serotonin. Note: Stevia is an acceptable sugar substitute. See page 4 for tips on how to eliminate sugar.

3. Eat more fish, especially wild, sustainable cold water varieties.

4. Eat lean meat from local organic, free-range or grass-fed animals.

5. Eat mostly high fiber, non-starchy vegetables and fruit. See page 5 for a list.

6. Use more spices and herbs to flavor foods instead of salt, sugar and fat.

7. Use only healthy oil for cooking. Olive, camelina, avocado, macadamia nut and coconut oil are anti-inflammatory fats. Food high in saturated fats, (ie. hamburgers, french fries, and other fried food) lead to sluggishness, slow thinking, fatigue, and poor circulation in the brain (eventually).

8. When thirsty, opt for water and herbal/non-caffeinated teas. Do not drink regular or diet pop.

9. Eat organic as much as you can, or follow the three rules:
   A. Buy corn, sugar, canola and soy in the organic form as these foods are genetically modified.
   B. The 'Dirty Dozen' list is the most heavily-sprayed foods that should be eaten organically.
   C. The 'Clean Fifteen' list is the least-sprayed foods that can be eaten non-organic. See list on page 6. These lists are updated annually by the Environment Working Group.

10. Identify and avoid food allergens - discuss testing with your Naturopathic Doctor.

11. Limit your intake of refined grains ie. white bread, white sugar, instant oats, white rice and instant noodles. Wheat gluten (a protein found in wheat) has been linked to depressive disorders.

12. Consider reducing your intake of dairy products by 50% and ensure the dairy products you consume are 100% organic. If you eat cheese, only eat white cheese.

13. Snack on unsalted nuts and seeds.

14. Consider eliminating caffeine or limit your intake to 6 oz per day. Caffeine can play a strong role in depression and anxiety.

15. Drink water/fluids between meals. Drink less during meals to avoid diluting digestive enzymes which compromises digestion. The minimum amount of water you need is 1/2 your body weight (lbs) in ounces.

16. Avoid skipping meals.

17. Eat tryptophan rich foods to help make serotonin: beef, chicken, turkey, tuna, salmon, cashews, peanuts, cottage cheese, avocado, tempeh, tofu, halibut, eggs, shrimp, lentils, quinoa, millet and oatmeal.

18. Avoid aspartame and other artificial sweeteners (eg. NutraSweet, Equal, Splenda) which are found in many diet sodas and sugar-free gums. Aspartame can block the formation of serotonin and cause headaches, insomnia, and depression in individuals who are already serotonin-deprived.

19. Prepare meals with and for others.

20. Eating healthy takes time and organization. Take the time to plan what you are going to make and what you need to buy (see shopping lists on pages 9-12). Allow enough time for meal preparation so you aren't rushed and tempted to reach for a quick fix. If you have a busy life, I suggest making meals in advance on the weekend and freezing ahead of time. I also recommend seeing what you can cut out of your life to create more time for a healthier you.

Tips on how to eliminate sugar:

Do you find that you can't get through the day without a sugary snack? You may be one of many people who are "addicted" to sugar. Sugar is the one substance that I have a bumpy relationship with - I eliminate it for months and then a chocolate occasion occurs (i.e. Valentine's Day, Easter) - and the next thing you know I am craving it again. The sugar roller coaster includes blood sugar crashes, headaches, mood swings, acne and weight gain - not very fun for my body, mind or spirit. When I was in the throes of my eating disorder, sugar became my "go-to drug" of choice. (You can read more about my mental health history in my book "Beyond the Label" available on Amazon.com).

Signs of sugar addiction include irritability, headaches, mood swings and insomnia. Sugar addiction is, in part, a by-product of sugar's purity – the body is not suited to accommodate this level of refinement. Simple sugars (i.e. white sugar, corn syrup) are refined to the point that digestion is practically superfluous.

When consumed, these sugars pass quickly into the bloodstream resulting in a temporary lift in energy. But, the sugar high leads to a sugar crash. This dangerous blood sugar roller coaster ride sets people up for future health problems, such as obesity, type 2 diabetes and cardiovascular problems. Simply providing the body with more sugar does not address the root problem. Underlying causes for sugar cravings include: low endorphin levels, hypoglycemia, endocrine imbalances, candida overgrowth and nutritional deficiencies.

In addition, sugar is an antidepressant of sorts. Consumption of sugar triggers the release of serotonin and dopamine, both of which are neurotransmitters involved in mental health. Sugar cravings are often a misguided attempt by the body to increase serotonin levels and thus elevate mood. The good news is that there are many other foods that increase serotonin levels without setting you up for long term health consequences like sugar.

• Withdraw slowly from sugar as quitting cold turkey can lead to restlessness, nervousness, headaches and depression. Watch a documentary on sugar (i.e. Fed Up, Hungry for Change). Increase your sugar awareness so you can decrease your sugar consumption.

• Remember your math: 4 grams is equal to 1 teaspoon of sugar.

• Eat within your limits. Determine what your average daily consumption of sugar is. From there, aim to have 1-2 less teaspoons of sugar per week until it is eliminated from your diet.

• Avoid processed junk food containing sugar: Sugar is an addictive substance that has an influence on dopamine, the pleasure neurotransmitter. When dopamine drops, we feel down. We crave this pleasant, feel-good feeling again...

so we reach for sugar and the cycle of addiction has begun. Break the cycle by avoiding processed junk food.

• Boost your serotonin: Serotonin can be raised by: following the dietary plan outlined in this book, daily exercise and adequate sleep. With sufficient serotonin, you crave sugar less.

• Use stevia to satisfy your sweet tooth: The all-natural sweetener, stevia, has 0 calories and does not raise blood sugar levels. Kick sugar cravings and satisfy your sweet tooth using stevia.

• Drink water: You may think your body needs sugar, when in fact it's dehydrated and really craving water!

• Stabilize blood sugar levels: Eat meals that support blood sugar levels by ensuring healthy fat, protein and complex carbohydrates (vegetables, whole grains and legumes) are included in your meals. Include a gluten-free grain, such as quinoa or millet at dinner so your body will produce more serotonin.

• Have plenty of greens: Nutrient-rich greens help boost your energy & reduce cravings for sugar.

• Eat sea vegetables: Sugar depletes minerals; restore them with mineral rich sea vegetables. Sprinkle dulse flakes on your salad, in soup or on an avocado.

• Consume more fermented foods and drinks: Try live fermented kefir, sauerkraut, kimchi, kombucha tea, natural plain yogurt and coconut kefir. You'll be amazed at how the sour taste of fermented foods and drinks quenches sugar cravings.

• Eat fresh fruit: Remind yourself that sugar is a dead energy food with no vitality. Compare that to biting into a juicy watermelon - there is no comparison! Enjoy the vitality of fresh fruit first to kick your craving for unhealthy sugary foods.

• Learn meditation & stress reduction techniques: Meditation can help ward off cravings by helping to reduce stress. Stress creates the hormone cortisol, which increases blood sugar levels. This is a vicious cycle that creates sugar cravings. Incorporate exercise, yoga or meditation into your routine to calm your body and mind.

• Try EFT (Emotional Freedom Technique): If you're looking to shift the desire for sugar, lose weight, stop a habit of binging or eliminate any addiction, consider EFT. EFT is an easy tool that anyone can learn in minutes. You simply tap on emotional acupressure points on your body while repeating key statements that help shift your body, mind and habits.

Referenced from: hungryforchange.tv/sugar-is-a-drug

List of non-starchy fruits and vegetables

The following is a list of non-starchy vegetables:

Amaranth or Chinese spinach
Artichoke hearts
Asparagus
Baby corn
Bamboo shoots
Beans (green, wax, Italian)
Bean sprouts
Beets
Brussels sprouts
Broccoli
Cabbage (green, bok choy, Chinese)
Cauliflower
Celery
Cucumber
Daikon
Eggplant
Greens (collard, kale, mustard, turnip)
Hearts of palm
Jicama

Kohlrabi
Leeks
Mushrooms
Okra
Onions
Pea pods
Peppers
Radishes
Rutabaga
Salad greens (chicory, endive, escarole, lettuce, romaine, spinach, arugula, radicchio, watercress)
Sprouts (broccoli, alfalfa)
Squash (summer, crookneck, spaghetti, zucchini)
Sugar snap peas
Swiss chard
Tomato
Turnips
Water chestnuts

Reference: diabetes.org

The following is a list of non-starchy fruits:

Watermelon
Cantaloupe
Grapefruit
Strawberries
Cranberries
Blackberries

Raspberries
Blueberries
Cherries
Pear
Plum
Apples

Reference: livestrong.com

Clean 15:

1. Sweet corn
2. Avocado
3. Pineapple
4. Cabbage
5. Onions
6. Sweet peas frozen
7. Papayas
8. Asparagus
9. Mangoes
10. Eggplant
11. Honeydew melon
12. Kiwi
13. Cantaloupe
14. Cauliflower
15. Grapefruit

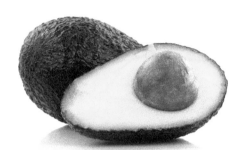

Dirty Dozen:

1. Strawberries
2. Spinach
3. Nectarines
4. Apples
5. Peaches
6. Pears
7. Cherries
8. Grapes
9. Celery
10. Tomatoes
11. Sweet bell pepper
12. Cucumber

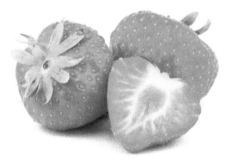

These lists are updated annually by the Environmental Working Group. See ewg.org

Dr. Chris's 2-Week Diet Plan and Recipes
for Nutritional Support of Balanced Mental Health

Week 1 Diet

	Mon.	Tues.	Wed.	Thurs.	Fri.	Sat.	Sun.
Breakfast	Steel cut oatmeal Non-dairy milk Organic pear	Warm quinoa porridge	Blueberry buckwheat pancakes	½ a cantaloupe Spelt toast w/ banana nut butter spread	Apple and hazelnut muesli	Crispy breakfast bars Blueberry hemp smoothie	½ a honeydew melon Poached or hard/soft boiled eggs Breakfast sausages
Morning Snack	Green goddess smoothie	Apple slices ¼ cup pumpkin seeds	Veggies w/ hummus	¼ cup unsalted nuts	¼ cup unsalted nuts	Organic celery sticks w/ almond butter	Brown rice cakes w/ almond butter
Lunch	Curried chicken salad Whole grain crackers	Lentil vegetable soup Cornmeal carrot muffin	Pita sandwich	Soba noodle veggie pot	Raw pad thai	Cranberry quinoa salad	Garden bean soup
Afternoon Snack	¼ cup unsalted nuts	¼ cup almonds	Organic fruit (1/2 - 1 cup)	Krispy kale chips	Veggies w/ Hummus	Organic fruit (1/2 - 1 cup)	Zucchini sticks w/ lentil dip
Dinner	Grilled salmon w/ balsamic onion glaze & steamed kale	Ginger chicken stir-fry	Turkey tacos	Three-bean vegetarian chili	Vegetable lasagna	Shrimp in Thai green curry w/ wild rice	Almond chicken Asian asparagus

Dr. Chris's 2-Week Diet Plan and Recipes
for Nutritional Support of Balanced Mental Health

Week 2 Diet

	Mon.	Tues.	Wed.	Thurs.	Fri.	Sat.	Sun.
Breakfast	Grain-free berry muffins Fresh fruit	Warm quinoa porridge	Berry-almond slam smoothie	Blueberry buckwheat pancakes	Instant flax cereal	Warm oat & apple bowl	Rice bread w/ sliced avocado
Morning Snack	¼ cup trail mix	Organic fruit (1/2 - 1 cup)	¼ cup unsalted nuts	Organic celery sticks w/ almond butter	¼ cup trail mix	Organic fruit (1/2 - 1 cup)	Organic celery sticks w/ almond butter
Lunch	Ginger butternut soup	Wonderful whatever salad (leftover chicken)	Warm spicy sweet potato salad	Edamame & bean salad w/ shrimp & fresh salsa	Salad rolls w/ tangy almond dipping sauce	Arugula rainbow salad	Garden bean soup
Afternoon Snack	Veggies w/ hummus	¼ cup almonds	Krispy kale chips	Apple slices handful of pumpkin seeds	Organic zucchini sticks w/ lentil dip	¼ cup trail mix	Organic fruit (1/2 cup - cup)
Dinner	Flax baked chicken Roasted beets & spinach salad	Vegetarian chili w/ avocado salsa	Sesame seed crusted salmon burgers w/ sliced avocado & Chickpea slaw	Spaghetti squash & black bean tacos	Almond chicken Stewed lentils & kale	Ultimate turkey & spinach lasagna	Pumpkin seed-crusted halibut & Kale salad

ESSENTIAL DIET GROCERY LIST : WEEK 1

PROTEINS
Rice, pea or hemp protein powder
8 boneless organic free range chicken breasts
4 turkey breasts
6 (4 oz) wild salmon fillets
2 C lentils
3 large eggs
3 (15 oz) cans chickpeas / garbanzo beans
2 lb. ground lean turkey
1 (15 oz) can pinto beans
1 (15 oz) can cannellini beans
1 (15 oz) can red kidney beans
1 lb. shrimp (fresh or frozen and defrosted)
4 oz silken organic tofu

LIQUIDS/DAIRY
1 L unsweetened almond, hemp or rice milk
1 C sour cream (optional)
1 (12 oz) can coconut milk 'not light'
½ C fresh apple juice

WHOLE GRAINS
1 box steel cut oats
1 rice pita
¾ C rolled quinoa flakes
3 C quinoa
1 C buckwheat flour
4 whole-wheat tortillas
1 package 100% buckwheat soba noodles
½ C rolled oats
1 pkg brown rice lasagna noodles
1 C wild rice

* Ensure organic as on "Dirty Dozen" list.

VEGGIES AND FRESH HERBS
2 bunches kale
2 bunches or bags fresh spinach*
1 bunch celery*
5 onions
6 large carrots*
16 garlic cloves
3 (28 oz) cans diced tomatoes
4 heads baby bok choy
2 (3-inch) pieces fresh ginger root
½ C sprouts
4 tomatoes*
1 bunch of lettuce
2 avocados
1 bunch scallions
2 sweet potatoes
1 head green or purple cabbage
1 butternut squash
1 bunch green onion
1 medium zucchini
1 large cauliflower floret
½ C mung bean sprouts or radish sprouts
2 limes or lemons
1 small eggplant
1 lb. mushrooms
1 red bell pepper*
1 ¼ C basil leaves
1 C chopped parsley
10-15 baby asparagus spears
1 bunch asparagus

FRUITS
1 pear*
1 C frozen strawberries*
1 fresh pineapple
1 C raisins
4 lemons
3 apples*
3 C blueberries
1 medium banana
½ C dried apricots
¾ C dried cranberries
¾ C dried blueberries

NUTS AND SEEDS
1 tbsp flax seed
¾ C raw almonds
1 jar tahini (sesame seed butter)
1 jar peanut butter
1 jar almond butter
2 ½ C fresh cashews
½ C hazelnuts
1 C pumpkin seeds
4 oz water chestnuts
¼ C sesame seeds
¾ C sunflower seeds
1 ½ C hemp seeds

OILS
Organic extra virgin olive oil
Organic canola oil
Coconut oil
Sunflower oil
Toasted sesame oil
Hemp seed oil
Sesame oil
Flaxseed oil

PANTRY
Stevia extract drops
Cinnamon
Raw honey
Brown sugar
Curry powder
Ground cornmeal
Chili powder
Chili pepper flakes or crushed red pepper flakes
Cardamom powder
1 jar Veganaise
Apple cider vinegar
Dijon mustard
Nutmeg powder
Teriyaki sauce
Turmeric
Parsley - fresh and dried

Balsamic vinegar
Baking soda
Baking powder
Pure vanilla extract
Cornstarch
Worcestershire sauce
1 L organic chicken broth
Nutritional yeast
Miso
Umeboshi plum paste
2 L organic vegetable broth
Maple syrup
Tamari
Thai Kitchen green curry paste
Thai Kitchen fish sauce
Paprika
Sea salt
Ground cumin
Ground oregano
Onion powder
Garlic powder
Dried basil
Ground pepper
Parsley fresh and dried
Ground sage
Ground savory
Ground ginger
Dried thyme
Garam masala (available at Indian grocery store)

PROTEINS

5 large organic eggs
2 C red split lentils
5 boneless organic free range chicken breasts
4 (15 oz) cans chickpeas
Rice, pea or hemp protein powder
1 (15 oz) can adzuki beans
1 Ib. wild salmon fillet
¼ C frozen shelled edamame
½ C small shrimp
1 can cannellini beans
1 (15 oz) can black beans
2 C green lentils or 1 (15 oz) can lentils
¾ Ib. ground lean turkey
1 lb halibut fillet

LIQUIDS/DAIRY

Unsweetened rice or almond milk
1 ½ C organic, vegan ricotta cheese
½ C shredded organic vegan mozzarella-like cheese
Butter

WHOLE GRAINS

2 tbsp brown rice flour
¾ C rolled quinoa flakes
2/3 C uncooked quick-cooking barley
Rice bread
¾ C buckwheat flour
8-10 crispy corn tacos
1 package thin rice vermicelli noodles
8 Vietnamese rice paper wrappers
2 tbsp steel cut oats
12 lasagna noodles

VEGGIES AND FRESH HERBS

11 onions
12 garlic cloves
2 butternut squash (7 C)
3 (3-inch) pieces fresh ginger root
½ C fresh parsley
Watercress (optional)
6 small beets
1 fennel bulb
2-3 bunches or bags of spinach leaves*
1 small shallot leafy lettuce
2 cucumbers*
1 scallion
2 seeded tomatoes*
2 red bell peppers*
Artichoke hearts (packed in water, not oil)
1 (4.5 oz) can chopped green chilies
Fresh cilantro
2 avocado
2 jalapeno peppers
3 medium sweet potatoes
3 red onions
1 yellow bell pepper*
4 bunches kale
6 carrots
1 head of red cabbage
Fresh snipped dill
8 cherry tomatoes*
1-2 Ib. spaghetti squash
8 leaves Boston Bibb lettuce
4 green onions
1 C fresh mint
½ C fresh basil
2 C arugula
1 ½ C broccoli florets
1 bunch of radish
1 (10 oz) pkg frozen spinach*
1 bunch celery*
2 (14.5 oz) cans diced tomatoes*
½ C kalamata olives

* Ensure organic as on "Dirty Dozen" list.

FRUITS

1 C raspberries
1 ½ C fresh or frozen organic blueberries
8 oz. raisins
1 C frozen mixed berries*
1 banana
¼ C golden raisins
Organic apple puree
6 limes
6 lemons
2 apples*

NUTS AND SEEDS

2 ½ C almond flour
Tahini (sesame seed butter)
16 oz. raw unsalted pumpkin seeds
8 oz. raw unsalted sunflower seeds
¾ C walnut halves / chopped walnuts
¼ C chopped almonds or hemp seeds
¼ C hemp seeds
Almond butter
1 C fresh cashews
¼ C sesame seeds
1 C almonds
1 tbsp ground flaxseed
6 tbsp raw flax seed

OILS

Organic extra virgin olive oil
Organic canola oil
Sunflower oil
Sesame oil
Hemp seed oil
Coconut oil

PANTRY

Baking soda
Sea salt
Cinnamon
Unpasteurized liquid honey
Pure vanilla extract
Ground nutmeg
Dried parsley
Dried paprika
Garlic powder
Turmeric
Ground pepper
Cardamom powder
Chili powder
Ground cumin
Dried oregano
Nutritional yeast
Panko (Japanese breadcrumbs)
Tamari
Olive oil cooking spray
Dried dill
Chili pepper flakes or crushed red pepper flakes
Ground flaxseed
Hot sauce (optional)
3 L organic vegetable broth
Dried basil
Low-sodium organic marinara sauce (3 C)
Garam masala (available at Indian grocery store)
Ground cayenne pepper

* Ensure are organic as on "Dirty Dozen" list.

Steel Cut Oatmeal
(Serves 2)

Ingredients:
1 C dry organic steel cut oats
non-dairy milk
3 cups of water
pear
cinnamon

Directions: Bring 3 cups water to a boil, add oats and reduce heat to medium and cook for 20-30 mins. Add cinnamon as oats finish cooking. Stir in non-dairy milk to taste and slice organic pear on top.

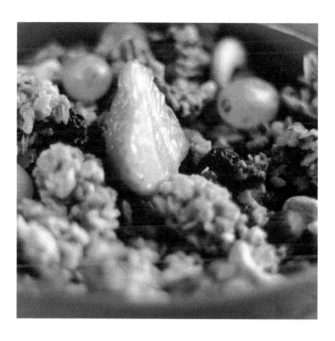

Green Goddess Smoothie
(Serves 1)

Ingredients:
1 C frozen organic strawberries
½ C diced fresh pineapple
1-3 kale leaves
1 handful of spinach leaves
1 to 2 C water, rice milk, or other milk substitute
1 serving protein powder that is as natural as possible without too many additives or intense flavours. Ask your ND for recommendations.
1 tbsp ground flaxseed or flaxseed oil

Directions: Put all ingredients in a food processor, magic bullet or blender and pulse until smooth, adding more liquid if necessary.

Curried Chicken Salad
(Serves 4+)

Ingredients:
2½ to 3 C (1 to 1.5 pounds) chicken or turkey, cooked, cooled, and diced
1 C diced organic celery
½ C organic raisins
½ C raw almond slices
1 to 2 tsp curry powder
¼ -½ tsp cayenne powder to taste
1 - 2 tsp apple cider vinegar
½ - 1 C mayonnaise or substitute (eg. Spectrum Naturals, Veganaise). See page 14 for Believable Vegan Mayonnaise recipe.

Directions: Combine the chicken, celery, raisins, and almond slices in a large bowl and mix together with a large spoon. Mix in curry and cayenne powder. Drizzle on the apple cider vinegar and add the mayonnaise, starting with ½ cup and adding more to your preference. Refrigerate for 1-2 hours before serving to enable flavors to integrate.

Believable Vegan Mayonnaise
Makes approximately ½ cup

Ingredients:
4 oz silken organic tofu
2 tsp fresh organic lemon juice
2 tsp Dijon mustard
1 C oil (olive, camelina hemp, flax or avocado oil)
sea salt

Directions: Combine tofu, lemon juice and mustard in a blender or with a wand blender for 30 seconds or until the tofu is smooth. While blending, slowly add in the oil and salt until emulsified and the mixture thickens to a mayonnaise-like consistency.

Steamed Kale
(Serves 4)

Ingredients:
1 bunch kale (stems removed), chopped
Juice of 1 lemon
2-3 tbsp olive oil
Pinch of sea salt

Directions: Steam kale until tender, approx. 3 min. Dress with lemon juice, olive oil and sea salt. Swiss chard and mustard greens can be prepared and dressed the same way.

Grilled Salmon with Balsamic Onion Glaze
(Serves 2)

Ingredients:
Balsamic Onion Glaze
2 tbsp olive oil
2 large onions, sliced
⅓ C balsamic vinegar
salt and pepper
Salmon
½ C balsamic vinegar
2 sprig fresh rosemary
6 x 4 oz wild salmon fillet portions, bones removed
olive oil
salt and pepper

Directions:
For balsamic onion glaze, heat oil in a large sauté pan over medium heat and add onions. Sweat onions, stirring often, until all liquid has evaporated, about 20 minutes. Add half the balsamic vinegar and simmer until absorbed. Add remaining balsamic vinegar and reduce until a glaze. Season to taste and set aside.

Salmon:
1. Preheat a grill to medium-high.
2. Reduce balsamic with rosemary in a small saucepot to a glaze consistency, about 8 minutes and set aside.
3. Brush salmon fillets lightly with olive oil and season. Grill skin-side up, for 4 minutes, then rotate 90 degrees and cook 4 more minutes.
4. Turn salmon over and cook for 8 more minutes for medium doneness. Brush salmon with rosemary balsamic mixture during last 5 minutes of cooking.
5. Serve salmon with Balsamic Onions on the side.

Warm Quinoa Porridge
(Serves 2)

Ingredients:
2 C filtered water
¾ C rolled quinoa flakes
1 tsp cinnamon
½ tsp cardamom powder
¼ tsp nutmeg
¼ tsp turmeric
1 tbsp raw honey OR 5 drops stevia extract liquid
pinch of sea salt
½ C apple, diced
½ C blueberries (if frozen add before quinoa to thaw)
¼ C chopped almonds or hemp seeds

Directions: Boil water in a small saucepan. Add the rolled quinoa flakes and stir for 2 to 3 minutes. Remove from heat and mix in the spices, raw honey, apple, blueberries and almonds.

Lentil Vegetable Soup
(Serves 6) *Prepare night before (2 hr prep)

Ingredients
2 C lentils
6 C filtered water
2 C organic chicken broth
½ C chopped onion
½ C chopped organic celery
¼ C chopped organic carrot
3 tbsp organic parsley
1 clove garlic
2 tsp salt
¼ tsp pepper
½ tsp oregano
1 tbsp Worcestershire sauce
1 x 28 oz can diced tomatoes
2 tbsp apple cider vinegar

Directions: Rinse lentils and place in a large soup pot. Add water and chicken broth and the remaining ingredients except tomatoes and apple cider vinegar. Cover and simmer for 1 ½ hours. Add tomatoes and vinegar and simmer for ½ hour more.

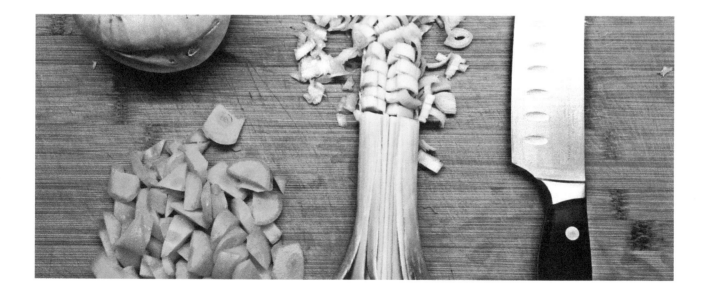

Cornmeal Carrot Muffins
(Makes 12)

Ingredients:
1 C flour blend-rice, quinoa, buckwheat etc.
¾ C coarsely ground cornmeal
1 tsp baking soda
1 tsp baking powder
½ tsp salt
½ C brown sugar
2 large eggs
½ C organic canola oil
½ C rice milk
1 ½ C grated carrots

Directions: Preheat oven to 350F. Line a 12-cup muffin tin with paper liners. Combine the flour blend, cornmeal, baking soda, baking powder, and salt in a medium bowl and set aside. Whisk the eggs and the brown sugar in a large bowl until frothy. Add the oil and milk and whisk to combine. Stir in the carrots and then mix in the dry mixture. Stir until no flour clumps remain. Divide the batter evenly between the muffin cups and bake 20 to 25 minutes. Cool 5 minutes, then transfer muffins to a wire rack to cool completely before serving.

Ginger Chicken Stir Fry
(Serves 2)

Ingredients:
4 baby bok choy
3 skinless, boneless organic free range chicken breasts
½ C teriyaki sauce
3 tbsp cornstarch
1 tsp grated fresh ginger
1 garlic clove
1 tbsp coconut oil
1 C organic, low sodium chicken broth
4 C spinach, lightly packed

Directions: Slice baby bok choy in half lengthwise. Cut chicken into bite-size strips. In a bowl, stir teriyaki and cornstarch until dissolved. Add garlic and ginger. Heat oil in a large frying pan or wok over medium-high heat. Add chicken and stir-fry until no longer pink, about 3 minutes. Add broth, teriyaki mixture and bok choy. Stir constantly until chicken is cooked, 3-4 minutes. Stir in spinach and serve over brown or wild rice.

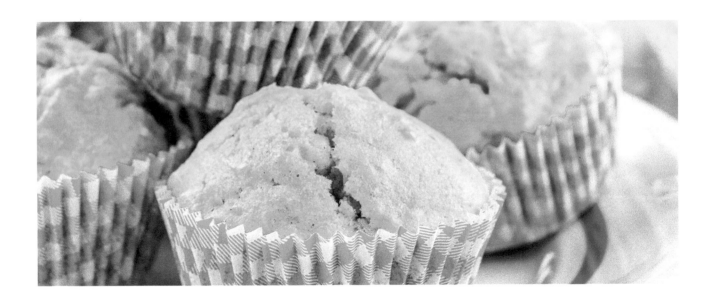

Blueberry Buckwheat Pancakes
(Serves 2)

Ingredients:
¾ C light or dark buckwheat flour
½ tsp cinnamon
¼ tsp sea salt
1 C fresh or frozen blueberries
3 tbsp unsweetened rice or almond milk
3 tbsp water
2 tbsp sunflower oil
½ tsp vanilla extract
1 flax egg replacer*
*To make the egg replacer, combine 1 tbsp of ground flaxseed with 3 tbsp of water and let sit for 2 minutes.

Directions: Stir the flour, cinnamon and salt together in a medium mixing bowl. Stir in the blueberries. Combine the milk, water, 1 tbsp of the sunflower oil, and the vanilla in a small bowl. Stir the flax egg replacer into the milk mixture. Pour the milk mixture into the flour mixture, mixing until just combined, using a whisk if necessary. If the batter is too stiff, more milk. Heat the remaining 1 tbsp of sunflower oil on a griddle or in a frying pan over medium-low heat, and then pour 2 tbsp of the batter onto the griddle, making 4 pancakes. Buckwheat flour browns quickly, so make sure the griddle or pan is not too hot. Once the edges are slightly browned and a few bubbles have formed on top, flip the pancakes over to cook the other side.

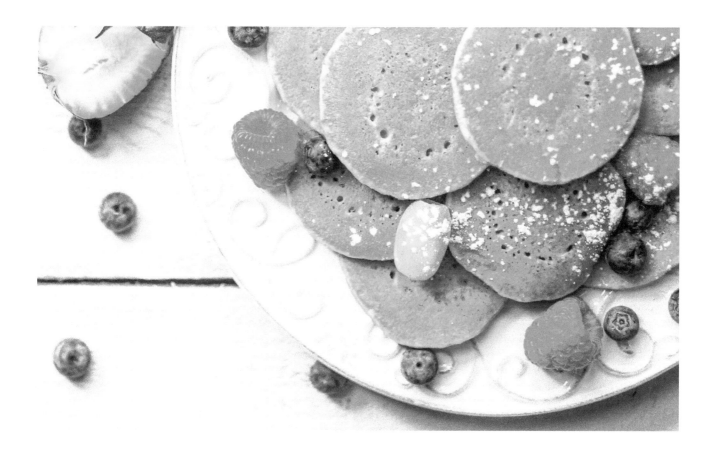

Pita sandwich
(Serves 1)

Ingredients:
1 medium rice pita
Turkey, sliced
Hummus (recipe below)
½ C sprouts
4 slices tomato
2-3 lettuce leaves

Directions: Slice one end of the pita so it creates a pouch. Spread hummus throughout the pita and fill pita with toppings.

Hummus
*Make enough to have as a snack tomorrow!
Makes 4 servings or approximately 1 cup

Ingredients:
1 15 oz can can chickpeas, rinsed and drained (save liquid)
2 garlic cloves, coarsely chopped
1 tbsp tahini (sesame seed butter)
Juice of 1 small lemon
1 tsp dried parsley
1 tsp paprika
½ tsp sea salt
1 tsp freshly ground pepper
¼ C extra-virgin olive oil

Directions: In a food processor, combine the chickpeas, garlic, tahini, lemon juice, parsley, paprika, salt and pepper. Pulse until combined. With the processor running, slowly add the olive oil through the feed tube, continually pulsing until mixture is smooth. If the hummus is still chunky, add some of the reserved chickpea liquid and process until hummus is smooth. Eat with your choice of organic veggies.

Turkey Tacos
(Serves 4)

Ingredients:
Jack's seasoning (recipe below)
1 tsp olive oil
1 lb. ground lean turkey
¾ C water
Whole-wheat tortillas
Optional: sour cream, avocado salsa (see recipe page 30), diced scallions, and tomatoes.

Directions: Heat the olive oil in a large skillet over medium-high heat. Break up the ground turkey into small pieces and cook thoroughly (5 minutes). Drain the fat and reduce the heat. Add the taco seasoning mix (recipe below) and water, then stir to blend the spices with the meat. Reduce the heat to simmer. Serve on a tortilla with diced scallions, tomatoes, sour cream and guacamole.

Jack's Taco Seasoning
(Serves 4)

Ingredients:
1 tsp ground cumin
1 tsp ground oregano
½ tsp onion powder
½ tsp garlic powder
½ tsp paprika
¼ to ½ tsp cayenne pepper (ground)
¼ to ½ tsp cayenne pepper flakes

Directions: Mix ingredients together, adding cayenne to taste.

Banana Nut Butter Spread
Makes ¾ -1 cup

Ingredients:
1 medium banana (can be frozen)
2-4 tbsp organic peanut butter, depending on taste (or almond, cashew, pumpkin seed butter, etc.)
½ tsp cinnamon
¼ tsp organic vanilla (optional)

Directions: Whisk ingredients in a food processor or blender until smooth. Leftovers can be stored in the fridge. Enjoy on gluten free toast with half a cantaloupe.

Krispy Kale Chips
(8 Cups)

Ingredients:
2 bunches green curly kale washed, large stem removed, torn into bite-sized pieces
"Cheese" Coating:
1 C unsalted cashews, soaked 2 hours
1 C sweet potato, grated
1 lemon, juiced (about 4 tbsp)
2 tbsp nutritional yeast
1 tbsp raw honey
½ tsp sea salt or pink rock salt
2 tbsp filtered water

Directions: Remove stems from kale and tear into bite-sized pieces. Place in large mixing bowl. Blend remaining ingredients in a blender until smooth. Pour over kale and mix thoroughly with your hands to coat (you want it to be really glued onto the kale.) Place kale onto unbleached parchment paper and dehydrate for 6 hours at 115 F. You'll need to use 2 trays. If you don't own a dehydrator, set your oven to 150 F and dehydrate for 2 hours. Turn leaves after 1 hour to ensure even drying. Remove and store in a dry, airtight container.

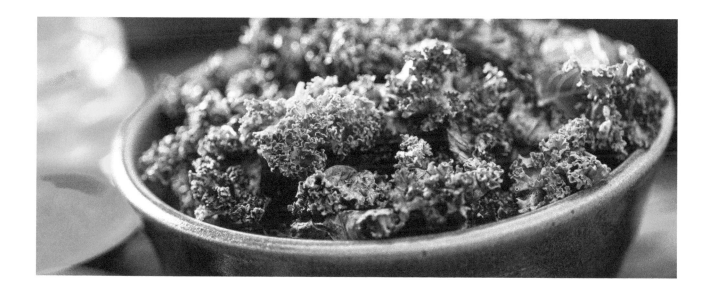

Soba Noodle Veggie Pot
(Serves 4)

Ingredients:
1 head green or purple cabbage
1 tbsp olive oil
1 C thinly sliced onion
1 C julienned carrot
1 tsp sea salt or pink rock salt, divided
½ package 100% buckwheat soba noodles
2 garlic cloves, minced

Dressing:
1 tbsp raw honey
2 tbsp miso
1 tbsp toasted sesame oil
½ C pumpkin seeds
½ tsp umeboshi plum paste (optional)

Directions: Slice cabbage into thin strips to make 3 cups (750 mL), set aside. Heat olive oil in a large skillet over medium-low heat, sauté onion until tender, about 5 minutes. Add cabbage, carrots and ½ tsp salt, stirring until cabbage is well coated. Reduce heat to medium-low. Cover and cook for 20 minutes stirring occasionally, until cabbage is very tender. Meanwhile, bring 4 L of filtered water to a boil in a large pot. Add the noodles and ½ tsp salt. Boil until al dente, about 6 minutes. Whisk dressing ingredients together and set aside. Drain noodles and rinse under warm running water. Toss noodles with the vegetable mixture and dressing. Serve and top with pumpkin seeds.

Three Bean Vegetarian Chili
(Serves 4)

Ingredients:
3 tbsp olive oil
1 C chopped onion
2 tsp ground cumin
1 tsp crushed red pepper
1 tsp paprika
¼ tsp salt
4 garlic cloves, thinly sliced
2 C organic vegetable broth
1½ C of ½-inch cubed peeled butternut squash
1 28 oz can diced tomatoes
1 15 oz can pinto beans, rinsed and drained
1 15 oz can cannellini beans, rinsed and drained
1 15 oz can red kidney beans, rinsed and drained
½ C thinly sliced green onion

Directions: Add oil to pan; swirl to coat. Add onion; cook 5 minutes, stirring occasionally. Stir in cumin, red pepper, paprika, salt and sliced garlic; cook 2 minutes; stirring frequently. Add broth, squash, and tomatoes; bring to a simmer. Cook 20 minutes, stirring occasionally. Add beans; simmer 25 minutes or until slightly thick, stirring occasionally. Sprinkle with green onions.

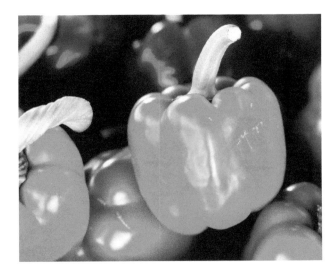

Apple and Hazelnut Muesli
(Serves 4)

Ingredients:
½ C rolled oats
½ C dried apricots, chopped
½ C toasted hazelnuts, chopped roughly
½ C fresh apple juice, ½ cup filtered water
2 apples, peeled and grated
1 tbsp maple syrup (optional)

Directions: In a large bowl mix together oats, apricots and hazelnuts. Add the apple juice and leave for 10 minutes to allow the oats and dried fruit to soak up the juice. Divide the muesli between 4 bowls and top with grated apple. Optional to drizzle maple syrup on top. Serve immediately.

Hummus
See Page 18 Week 1 Wednesday

Raw Pad Thai
(Serves 2-4)

Ingredients :
1 medium zucchini
1 large carrot
1 green onion, chopped
½ C shredded purple cabbage
½ C cauliflower florets
½ C mung beans sprouts or radish sprouts (spicy)

Sauce:
2 tbsp tahini
2 tbsp almond butter
1 tbsp lime or lemon juice
2 tbsp tamari (wheat-free)
1 tbsp raw honey
¼ tsp garlic, minced
½ tsp ginger root, grated

Directions: Use a spiralizer, mandolin or vegetable peeler to create noodles from carrots and zucchini. Place them in a large mixing bowl and top with the vegetables. Whisk sauce ingredients in a bowl. The sauce will be thick, but will thin out after its mixed with the vegetables. Pour the sauce over the noodles and vegetables, and toss. This dish tastes even better the next day once the flavors have had a chance to blend.

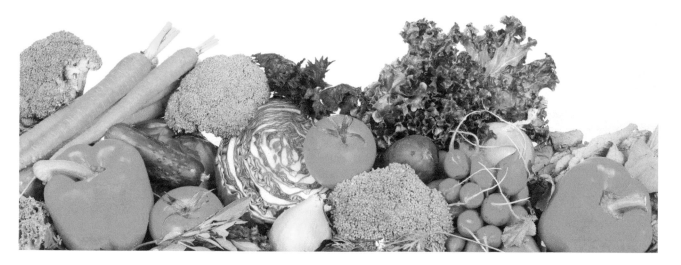

Vegetable Lasagna
(Serves 8)

Ingredients:
1½ C raw cashews
Sea salt
12 brown rice lasagna noodles
2 x ¼ C olive oil
1 white or yellow onion, diced
1 small eggplant, peeled and diced
1 lb. mushrooms, cleaned and sliced
1 red bell pepper, seeded and chopped
4 cloves garlic, minced-divided use
28 oz can diced tomatoes
½ tsp black pepper
¼ tsp crushed red pepper flakes
2 tsp dried basil
2 tsp dried oregano
1 tsp fresh lemon juice
2 tsp nutritional yeast
1 C fresh basil leaves
Directions: Soak cashews in filtered water for 2-24 hrs. Drain and set aside. Boil water in a large pot and cook the lasagna noodles according to the package directions. Drain and rinse noodles with hot water, drizzle with 1 tbsp olive oil and gently stir to coat the noodles. Set aside. In a large skillet heat 2 tablespoons olive oil over medium-high heat. Add the onion, eggplant, mushroom and red pepper. Cook the vegetables, stirring occasionally, until brown (15 min). Add 2 minced garlic cloves and cook for 30 seconds. Lower heat to medium, add tomatoes with their juice, 1 tsp salt, black pepper, red pepper flakes, dried basil and oregano and cook until most of the tomato liquid has reduced and the mixture is thick and cooked through.

Preheat oven to 350F. Place the soaked cashews in a blender with 1/3 cup water, the remaining 2 minced garlic cloves, lemon juice and nutritional yeast. Blend until smooth, scraping down the sides of the blender as needed. If needed, add more water, a little at a time. Remove half the mixture and reserve. To the remaining cashew cheese, add the fresh basil and remaining ¼ cup of olive oil and blend until smooth. Ladle a little of the liquid from the tomato vegetable mixture on the bottom of a 9x12 inch baking dish then layer half the lasagna noodles. Add half of the tomato vegetable mixture and top with the basil cashew cheese. Layer on the remaining lasagna noodles, the rest of the tomato vegetable mixture and then drizzle the top with the reserved cashew cheese. Bake uncovered until hot and bubbly, 30-40 minutes.

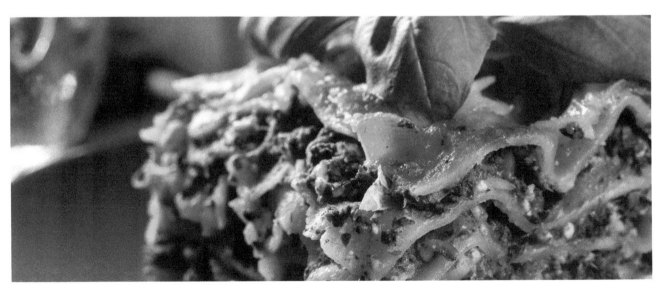

Crispy Breakfast Bars
(16 bars)

Ingredients:
7 C crispy puffed rice whole-grain cereal
¾ C dried cranberries
¾ C dried blueberries
½ C sunflower seeds
1 tsp cinnamon
¾ C brown rice syrup or honey
¾ C almond butter
2 tbsp coconut oil

Directions: Stir together puffed rice or cereal, dried fruit, sunflower seeds and cinnamon in a large bowl. Place syrup, almond butter, and coconut oil in a large pot. Heat on stove until almond butter has melted. Stir well and pour over cereal mixture. Stir to coat. Dampen your hands with cold water. Press cereal mixture firmly into a 9-inch square baking pan, rewetting hands if necessary to keep mixture from sticking. Freeze 30 minutes. Cut into 16 bars and store in refrigerator.

Cranberry Quinoa Salad
(Serves 6)

Ingredients:
2 C cooked quinoa
½ C hemp seeds
1 C chopped parsley
1 coarsely grated carrot
3 tbsp pumpkin seeds
3 tbsp dried cranberries

Dressing:
2 tsp hemp seed oil
2 tbsp lemon juice
1 tsp raw honey
½ tsp sea salt

Directions: Combine all salad ingredients in a large bowl. Combine all dressing ingredients in a small glass jar with a tight-fitting lid, and shake well. Toss the salad and dressing and serve immediately.

Blueberry Hemp Smoothie
(Makes 2.5 cups)

Ingredients:
2 tbsp hemp seeds
1 C fresh or frozen blueberries
½ C unsweetened almond, rice or hemp milk
½ C filtered water
1 tsp pure vanilla extract
½ tsp cinnamon
1 scoop protein powder (optional)

Directions: Put all ingredients into blender or magic bullet and blend until smooth. Ask your ND for a protein powder recommendation.

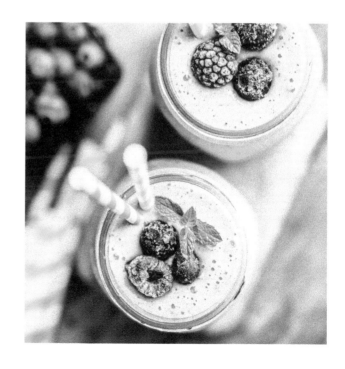

Shrimp in Thai Green Curry
(Serves 4)

Ingredients:
1 tbsp coconut oil
2-3 cloves garlic, sliced thinly
10-15 baby asparagus spears
1 12 oz can coconut milk (not light)
1 tbsp Thai Kitchen green curry paste
½ tsp turmeric
½ tsp red pepper flakes
1 lb shrimp, fresh or frozen and defrosted
½ tsp Thai Kitchen fish sauce (optional)
¼ C fresh basil leaves

Directions: Heat coconut oil in a deep skillet over high heat. When hot, sauté the garlic and asparagus until a little soft. Slowly pour the coconut milk into the skillet and then add the Thai Kitchen green curry paste, turmeric and red pepper flakes. Using a spatula, thoroughly mix the paste into the coconut milk, while bringing it to a light boil. Add the shrimp and fish sauce, if using. Cover the skillet (use aluminum foil if you don't have a lid), turn the heat down to medium, and cook for 10 minutes, stirring occasionally. Add the basil leaves and cook for 1 minute. Serve with wild rice, either plain or see wild rice recipe.

Wild Rice
(Serves 4)

Ingredients:
1 C wild rice
1 C organic vegetable broth
2 C water
2 stalks celery, diced
4 oz water chestnuts, diced
2 to 3 tbsp organic raisins

Directions: Rinse the rice in a strainer and transfer it to a pot. Add the broth and water. Bring to a boil over high heat, then cover and reduce heat to simmer. After 20 minutes, add the celery, water chestnuts and raisins to the rice and stir. The rice should be fully cooked in 40-50 minutes. Fluff it with a fork and drain off any excess liquid.

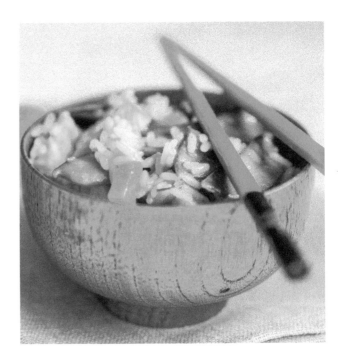

Breakfast Sausages
(Makes 9)

Ingredients:
1 lb (455 g) ground turkey
1 egg lightly beaten (optional)
1 tsp ground sea salt
½ tsp ground sage
¼ tsp ground savory
⅛ tsp ground nutmeg
⅛ tsp ground ginger
¼ tsp black pepper
3 shakes cayenne pepper
2 shakes dried thyme
1 ½ tsp olive oil
¾ tsp honey

Directions: Place ground meat in a large bowl, add egg and mix in well. Combine salt and seasonings in a separate bowl. Sprinkle seasoning over the meat and work in until blended evenly. Drizzle the olive oil and honey over the meat and work in. Shape into nine patties and fry at medium heat, covered. Turn frequently and watch closely. Cook for approximately 10-15 minutes.

Garden Bean Soup
(Serves 8)

Ingredients:
1 tsp olive oil
2 onions, chopped
1 C chopped celery
1 C diced carrots
2 tsp grated fresh ginger
1 tsp minced garlic
1 tsp garam masala (available at an Indian grocery store)
1 tsp turmeric
½ tsp ground cumin
¼ tsp ground cayenne pepper
6 C organic vegetable broth
1 C lentils, uncooked
2 x 15 oz cans garbanzo beans, rinsed and drained
1 x 14 oz can diced tomatoes, undrained

Directions: Pour olive oil into a large soup pot set over medium-high and sauté onions 3 to 4 minutes or until tender. Add carrots and celery and cook for 5 minutes. Stir in minced garlic, ginger and spices and cook for 30 seconds. Add broth and remaining ingredients and cook until lentils are tender, about 90 minutes. If desired, half of the soup can be pureed and stirred back into the pot for a thicker, creamier soup.

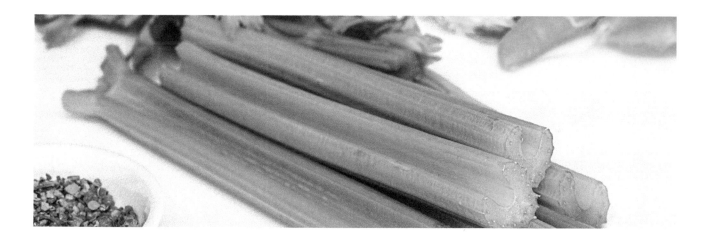

Almond Chicken
(Serves 2)

Ingredients:
½ C ground almonds
1 tbsp dried oregano
1 tsp dried basil
1 tbsp dried parsley
½ tsp sea salt
1 tsp freshly ground pepper
2 tbsp olive oil
2 boneless, skinless chicken breasts

Directions: Preheat the oven to 450 F. Combine the almonds, oregano, basil, parsley, salt and pepper in a small bowl. Rinse the chicken breasts and pat dry with paper towels and place on a plate. Gently pat the chicken on each side with the almond mixture and place on a baking sheet or in a shallow glass-baking dish. Drizzle the olive oil over the chicken and bake for 12 to 15 minutes, depending on the thickness of each breast.

Asian Asparagus
(Serves 2 - 4)

Ingredients:
1 bunch of asparagus
½ C water
1 tbsp sesame oil
1 tsp sunflower oil
1 tsp freshly ground pepper
½ tsp sea salt
2 tbsp sesame seeds

Directions: Wash asparagus, break off the hard ends. Put the asparagus and water in a large sauté pan and place on the stove over medium-high heat. Cover and steam for 3 minutes. Uncover, reduce the heat to low and add the sesame and sunflower oils, salt, pepper, and sesame seeds. Stir to coat and cook, uncovered, for another 5 minutes.

Lentil Dip
(See Page 35 Week 2 Friday)

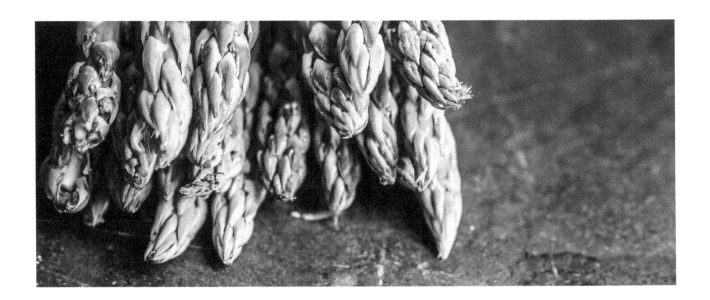

Grain-Free Berry Muffins
(Yields 12 muffins)

Ingredients:
2 ½ C almond flour
1 tsp baking soda
½ tsp sea salt
1 tbsp cinnamon
½ C olive oil
3 large organic eggs
½ C unpasteurized liquid honey
1 tbsp pure vanilla extract
1 C organic blueberries or raspberries, fresh or frozen

Directions: Preheat oven to 300 F. Line a standard 12-cup muffin tin with paper liners. In a medium bowl, whisk together the almond flour, baking soda, salt and cinnamon. Add the oil, eggs, honey and vanilla to the dry ingredients and stir until the batter is smooth. Gently fold in the blueberries just until they are evenly distributed throughout the batter. Divide the batter between muffin cups. Bake on the center rack for 35 minutes, rotating the pan after 15 minutes. A toothpick inserted into the center of the muffin should come out clean. Let the muffins stand for 15 minutes, then transfer to a wire rack and let cool completely. Store the muffins in an airtight container at room temperature for up to 3 days.

Trail Mix
(Makes ¾ cup)

Ingredients:
4 oz unsalted pumpkin seeds
4 oz unsalted sunflower seeds
4 oz raisins

Directions: Combine and store in a container in the refrigerator to avoid rancidity if storing for long periods of time.

Ginger Butternut Soup
(Serves 6)

Ingredients:
2 C finely chopped onions
1 tbsp olive oil
2 garlic cloves. minced
10 C (2.5 L) filtered water or vegetable stock
7 C (1.75 L) butternut squash, peeled and diced
1 C red split lentils
1 tbsp minced fresh ginger root OR ½ teaspoon powdered ginger root
1 tsp ground cinnamon
¼ tsp ground nutmeg
3 tbsp tahini
1 tsp sea salt
parsley or watercress (optional)

Directions: In a large soup pot over medium-low heat, cook the onion in the oil about 2 to 3 minutes, until the onions are translucent. Stir in minced garlic, add squash, lentils, and water or stock. Cover and bring to a boil over high heat. Uncover pot and skim off lentil foam with a spoon. Reduce heat and simmer until the squash and lentils are tender, about 40 minutes. Using a blender, food processor or immersion blender, puree the squash mixture along with the spices, tahini and salt. Serve hot, garnished with roasted pumpkin or squash seeds and parsley or watercress, if desired.

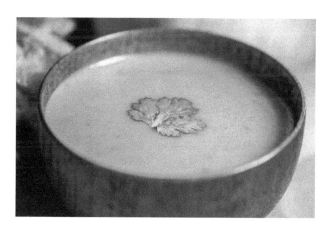

Flax Baked Chicken
(Serves 2)

Ingredients:
2 tbsp brown rice flour
1 tbsp ground flaxseed
1 tsp dried parsley
1 tsp dried paprika
1 tsp garlic powder
½ tsp turmeric
½ tsp sea salt
1 tsp freshly ground pepper
2 boneless, skinless chicken breasts
3 tbsp olive oil

Directions: Preheat oven to 450 F. In a small mixing bowl, combine the flour, flaxseed, parsley, paprika, garlic powder, turmeric, salt and pepper. Place the flour mixture in a Ziploc bag. Rinse and pat the chicken breasts dry. Coat the breasts with olive oil. Put the chicken in the bag with the flour mixture and thoroughly coat each piece. Place the chicken on a baking sheet or shallow glass-baking dish and bake for 12 to 15 minutes, depending on the thickness of the chicken.

Hummus
See Page 18 Week 1 Wednesday

Roasted Beets and Spinach Salad
(Serves 2)

Ingredients:
6 small beets, boiled and quartered
1 fennel bulb, tops cut off and bulb quartered
2 tbsp plus ¼ cup olive oil
4 C loosely packed baby spinach leaves
1 small avocado, peeled and diced
1 small shallot, minced
Juice of half a lemon
½ tsp sea salt
½ tsp freshly ground pepper
½ C walnut halves, toasted

Directions: Preheat the oven to 450 F. Place the beets and fennel on a baking sheet, drizzle with 2 tbsp of olive oil, and roast in the oven for 15 minutes. Meanwhile, combine the spinach and avocado in a mixing bowl. To make the dressing, put the shallot, lemon juice, salt, pepper and the ¼ cup of olive oil in a small food processor and pulse for 1 minute. Toss the dressing with the spinach and avocado and place on two serving plates. Place half the roasted beets and fennel on each plate and sprinkle the walnuts over each serving.

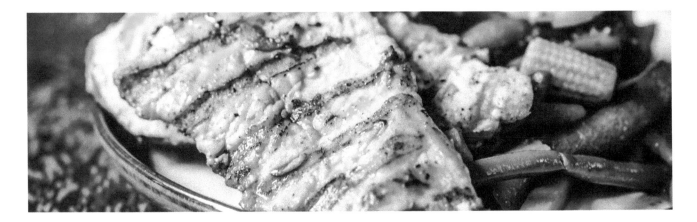

Warm Quinoa Porridge
(Serves 2)

Ingredients:
2 C filtered water
¾ rolled quinoa flakes
1 tsp cinnamon
½ tsp cardamom powder
¼ tsp nutmeg
¼ tsp turmeric
1 tbsp raw honey
⅛ tsp sea salt
½ C organic apple, diced
½ C blueberries (if frozen, add before quinoa to thaw)
¼ C chopped almonds or hemp seeds

Directions: Boil water in a small saucepan. Add the rolled quinoa and stir for 2 to 3 minutes. Remove from heat and mix in the spices, raw honey, apple, blueberries and almonds or hemp seeds.

Wonderful Whatever Salad
(Serves 1)

Ingredients:
Any green leafy lettuce (not iceberg) or spinach
Cucumber
Scallion, diced
Tomato or bell peppers
Sliced almonds
Artichoke hearts (packed in water, not oil)
Hemp nut seeds
Flax baked chicken, leftover from night before

Directions: Prepare the ingredients in the desired amounts and toss with any dressing!

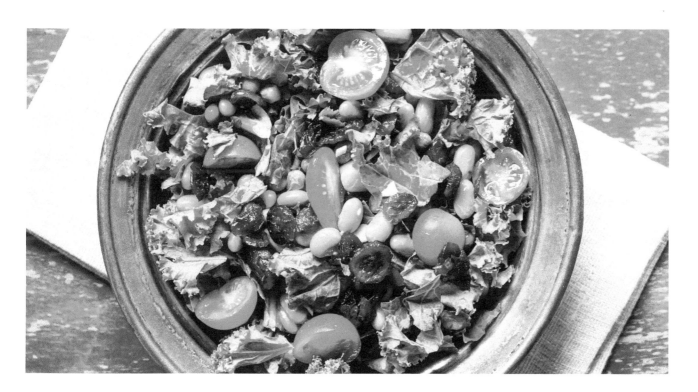

Vegetarian Chili
(Serves 6)

Ingredients:
2 tsp organic canola oil
1 C chopped onion
1 C chopped red bell pepper
2 tsp chili powder
1 tsp ground cumin
1 tsp dried oregano
3 garlic cloves, minced
1 x 4.5 oz can chopped green chilies
⅔ C uncooked quick-cooking barley
¼ C water
1 x 15 oz can diced tomatoes, undrained
2 C vegetable broth
3 tbsp chopped fresh cilantro
6 lime wedges
18 baked organic tortilla chips

Directions: Heat the oil over medium-high heat. Add onion and bell pepper; sauté 3 minutes. Add chili powder and next 4 ingredients (chili powder through green chilies); cook 1 minute. Stir in barley and next 4 ingredients (barley through broth); bring to a boil. Cover, reduce heat, and simmer for 20 minutes or until barley is tender. Stir in cilantro. Serve with lime wedges, chips and Avocado Salsa.

Avocado Salsa
(Makes 1 cup)

Ingredients:
½ C finely chopped avocado
⅓ C chopped seeded tomato
2 tbsp finely chopped onion
1 tbsp finely diced seeded jalapeno pepper
1 tbsp chopped fresh cilantro
1 tbsp fresh lime juice
⅛ tsp salt

Directions: Combine all ingredients; toss.

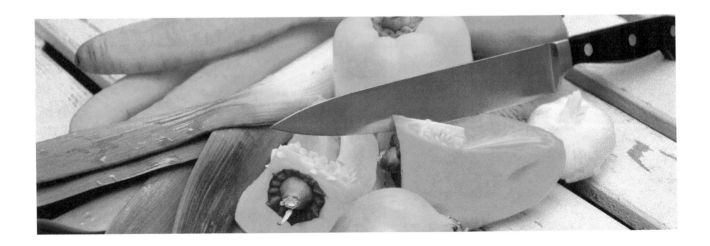

Berry-Almond Slam Smoothie
(Serves 1)

Ingredients:
1 ½ C frozen mixed organic berries (strawberries, blueberries, and raspberries)
1 ½ C almond milk
1 tbsp almond butter
1 serving protein powder

Directions: Put all ingredients in a food processor or blender and pulse until smooth, adding more liquid if necessary. Ask your ND for a protein powder recommendation.

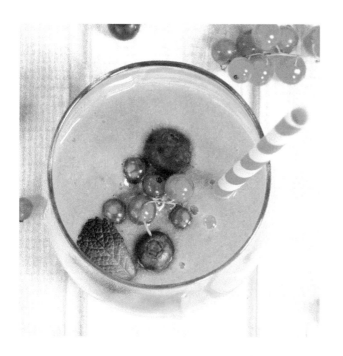

Warm Spicy Sweet Potato Salad
(Serves 4)

Ingredients:
2 medium sweet potatoes, diced
1 small red onion, diced
1 tbsp plus ¼ cup olive oil
1 C loosely packed, chopped fresh cilantro
1 x 15 oz can adzuki beans, drained and rinsed
1 organic yellow bell pepper, seeded and diced
1 garlic clove, coarsely chopped
1 jalapeno pepper seeded
Juice of 1 lime
½ tsp sea salt
½ tsp freshly ground pepper

Directions: Preheat the oven to 450 F. Place the sweet potatoes and onion on a baking sheet and drizzle with the 1 tbsp of olive oil to coat. Roast in oven for 25 minutes. While the sweet potatoes are roasting, toss the cilantro, beans and the bell pepper in a small bowl.

To make the dressing, combine the garlic, jalapeno pepper, lime, salt and pepper in a small food chopper or processor. Process for 10 seconds, and then add ¼ cup olive oil and continue to process for another minute. Toss the roasted sweet potatoes and onion with the bean mixture and pour the dressing over top. Combine to thoroughly coat and serve warm.

Krispy Kale Chips
See Page 19 Week 1 Thursday

Sesame Seed-Crusted Salmon Burgers
(Serves 4)

Ingredients:
1 (1-lb) wild salmon fillet, skinned and chopped
2 C chopped baby spinach
¼ C Panko (Japanese breadcrumbs)
1 tbsp fresh lemon juice, divided
1 tbsp tamari
¼ C sesame seeds, toasted and divided
¼ tsp salt
¼ tsp black pepper
Olive oil cooking spray

Directions: Combine salmon, spinach, Panko, lemon juice, tamari, 1 tbsp sesame seeds, salt and pepper in a large bowl. Form mixture into 4 (3 ½ -inch) patties. Place remaining sesame seeds onto a plate, and dip one side of patties into seeds to coat. Preheat a lightly oiled grill pan over medium heat until hot but not smoking. Cook burgers over medium heat, turning, 3-4 minutes per side or until golden brown and cooked through.

Chickpea Slaw
(Serves 4)

Ingredients:
2 medium carrots, peeled and shredded
1 small bunch of kale, shredded
½ small head of red cabbage, shredded
1 x 15 oz can chickpeas, drained and rinsed
2 tbsp pumpkin seeds
1 tsp dried dill or 1 tbsp snipped fresh dill
1 tsp dried oregano or 1 tbsp chopped fresh oregano
½ tsp sea salt
½ tsp freshly ground pepper
½ tsp chili pepper flakes
½ C olive oil
Juice of 1 lemon

Directions: Mix the carrots, kale, cabbage, chickpeas, and pumpkin seeds in a serving bowl and set aside. To make the dressing, combine the dill, oregano, salt, chili pepper flakes and pepper in a small bowl. Add the olive oil and lemon juice and whisk until blended well. Pour the dressing over the slaw, tossing to coat evenly.

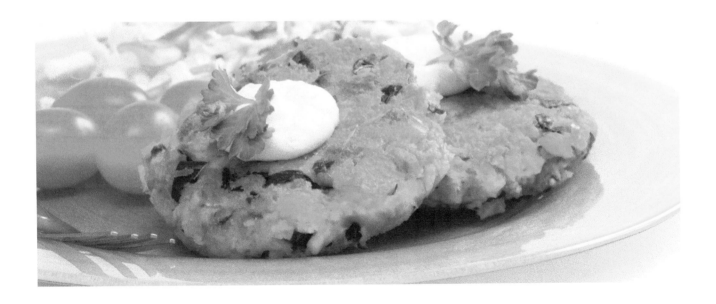

Week 2 Thursday

Blueberry Buckwheat Pancakes
See Page 17 Week 1 Wednesday

Spaghetti Squash and Black Bean Tacos
(Serves 4)

Ingredients:
1-2lb spaghetti squash (if you go bigger, increase spices accordingly)
Juice of 1 lime (about 2 tbsp)
1 tsp chili powder
1 tsp sea salt
1 tsp garlic powder
1 14 oz can black beans, thoroughly rinsed
8-10 crispy organic corn tacos
Cilantro
Hot sauce (optional)

Directions: Preheat oven to 400 F. Cut spaghetti squash in half lengthwise, scoop out the seeds, spread 1 tsp olive oil on each half and roast both halves face down on a rimmed baking sheet until tender and easily pierced with a fork, 45-60 minutes. Meanwhile, combine lime juice, chili powder, salt, cumin and garlic powder in a small bowl. When spaghetti squash is done remove from oven and let cool until you can handle it easily. Working over a large bowl, gently scrape out the flesh with a fork. Add lime mixture to the squash and toss well to combine. In the bottom of each corn taco, spread 2 tbsp of black beans. Top with spaghetti squash. Line the tacos in a 9X13 baking dish and bake in preheated oven for 20 minutes. To serve, top with fresh cilantro and hot sauce if desired.

Edamame and Bean Salad with Shrimp and Fresh Salsa
(Serves 4)

Ingredients:
¼ C frozen shelled edamame
½ C chopped cooked small shrimp (about 3 ounces)
½ C canned cannellini beans, rinsed and drained
½ C halved cherry tomatoes
1 to 2 tbsp chopped red onion
1 tsp minced jalapeno pepper
1 tbsp chopped fresh cilantro
2 tsp fresh lime juice
1 ½ tsp olive oil
⅛ tsp salt

Directions: Cook edamame according to package directions. Drain and rinse with cold water; drain. Combine edamame, shrimp, cannellini beans, cherry tomatoes, onion and jalapeno pepper. Combine cilantro and the remaining ingredients, stirring with a whisk. Drizzle over edamame mixture and toss gently to combine. Cover and chill.

Fresh Salsa
(Serves 4)

½ C halved cherry tomatoes
1 to 2 tbsp chopped red onion
1 tsp minced jalapeno pepper
1 tbsp chopped fresh cilantro
2 tsp fresh lime juice
1 ½ tsp olive oil
⅛ tsp salt

Combine cilantro and the remaining ingredients, stirring with a whisk. Drizzle over edamame mixture and toss gently to combine. Cover and chill.

Instant Flax Cereal
(Serves 1)

Ingredients:
6 tbsp flax seeds
4 to 8 oz non-dairy milk (hemp, almond, rice)
½ banana, sliced

Directions: Grind flax seeds to a powder using a coffee or seed grinder. Place powder in a cereal bowl and slowly add non-dairy milk, stirring the mixture together. The flax mixture will thicken into a cereal with a texture similar to cream of rice. Top cereal with sliced bananas. Eat the mixture right away because the flax seeds are sensitive to light, air and temperature. Eat it cold. Do not cook this cereal.

Trail Mix
See Page 27 Week 2 Monday

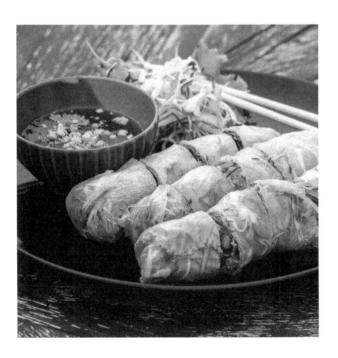

Fresh Salad Rolls
(Serves 4)

Ingredients:
8 leaves of Boston Bibb lettuce
2 carrots, peeled and julienned
½ organic cucumber, peeled and julienned
3 green onions, thinly sliced, white and pale green parts only
1 C loosely packed, chopped fresh cilantro
1 C loosely packed, chopped fresh mint
1 C finely chopped almonds
½ package thin rice vermicelli noodles, cooked
8 Vietnamese rice paper wrappers

Directions: The easiest way to put together the salad rolls is to make an assembly line on the kitchen countertop or table, starting with the lettuce leaves. Fill a large bowl with warm water. Submerge 1 rice paper wrapper in the water for 10 seconds, or just until it becomes soft. Remove the wrapper to a flat work surface, and let it rest for 30 seconds; it will become easier to handle.

Place 1 leaf of lettuce just below the middle of the wrapper, leaving a 1-inch border on each side. Top with ¼ cup of the noodles, then 2 or 3 slices of the cucumber and carrots. Sprinkle a few green onions and cilantro and mint on the veggies, then top with some of the almonds.

Fold the bottom of the wrapper up over the filling pressing the filling as you go. Fold both sides of the wrapper inward. Gently press to seal and roll the wrapper to the top edge. Repeat with the remaining wrappers. Serve with tangy almond dipping sauce (See page 35).

Tangy Almond Dipping Sauce
(Makes 3/4 cup)

Ingredients:
1 piece of fresh ginger, chopped
1 garlic clove, chopped
2 tbsp almond butter
Juice of 1 lime
1 tsp chili pepper flakes
1 ½ tsp sesame oil
½ C water, or more as needed
¼ tsp sea salt

Directions: In a food processor or blender, mince the ginger and garlic. Add the almond butter, lime juice, and chili pepper flakes and blend. Lastly, add the sesame oil, water and salt and blend until smooth.

Lentil Dip
(Makes 3 cups)

Ingredients:
1 x 15 oz canned lentils, drained or 2 cups cooked lentil
1 C almond butter or chopped walnuts
2 tbsp hemp seed oil
1 large garlic clove
½ cup fresh basil
⅓ C lemon juice
1 tsp lemon zest
1 tsp turmeric
¼ tsp sea salt

Directions: Process all ingredients in a food processor fitted with an S-blade. Blend until very smooth. Serve with zucchini sticks.

Stewed Kale and Lentils
(Serves 4)

Ingredients:
1 tbsp olive oil
1 red onion, chopped
3 cloves garlic, minced
1 tbsp minced fresh ginger
1 carrot, peeled and diced
½ tsp ground cumin
½ tsp cinnamon
1 C dried green lentils
3 C organic vegetable broth
4 C chopped, stemmed kale
¼ C golden raisins
¼ C chopped walnuts, toasted

Directions: Heat oil over medium heat; cook onion, garlic and ginger, stirring occasionally, until softened, about 5 minutes. Add carrot, cumin and cinnamon; cook, stirring occasionally, until fragrant, about 3 minutes. Stir in lentils to coat. Add broth and bring to boil; reduce heat, cover and simmer until lentils are al dente, about 10 minutes. Add kale and raisins; simmer, covered, until lentils are tender, about 10 minutes. Uncover and cook until almost no liquid remains, about 4 minutes. Sprinkle with toasted walnuts.

Almond Chicken
(Serves 2)
See Page 26 Week 1 Sunday

Warm Oat and Apple Bowl
(Serves 1)

Ingredients:
2 tbsp olive oil or coconut oil
2 tbsp steel-cut oats
1 tbsp organic apple puree (no sugar added)
2 tsp flaked almonds
2 tsp pumpkin seeds
2 tsp ground almonds

Directions: Heat oil gently in a small saucepan. Add the oats and stir until starting to go golden. Add remaining ingredients and stir until starting to go golden. Add rest of ingredients and stir until heated through. Put in a bowl.

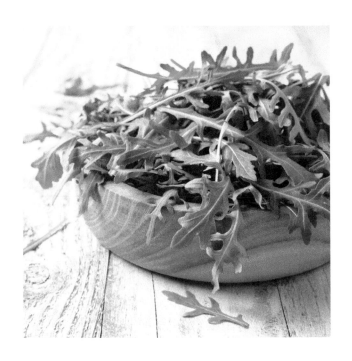

Arugula Rainbow Salad
(Serves 2)

Ingredients:
2 C arugula, torn into large pieces
1 ½ C broccoli florets
1 C coarsely grated carrot
½ C radish, finely diced
1 tbsp red onion, minced
3 oz (90 g) cooked chicken breast (optional)

Directions: Place arugula, broccoli, carrot, radish and onion in a medium bowl. Top with dressing of choice. Add chicken if including.

Trail Mix
See Page 27 Week 2 Monday

Ultimate Turkey and Spinach Lasagna
(Makes 9 Servings)

Ingredients:
1 tbsp olive oil
1 medium onion, chopped
2 minced garlic cloves
¾ lb ground free-range turkey breast
3 C low-sodium organic marinara sauce
1.5 C organic, vegan ricotta cheese
1 x 10 oz package frozen spinach, defrosted and squeezed of all excess liquid
¼ C chopped parsley
2 egg whites
¼ tsp salt
¼ tsp pepper
12 lasagna noodles, cooked al dente according to the package instructions
½ C shredded organic vegan mozzarella-like cheese

Directions: Preheat oven to 375F. Heat oil in a large high-sided skillet and cook onion, stirring occasionally, until softened, 6-7 minutes. Add garlic and cook 1 minute. Add turkey and cook, breaking up with a spoon, until no longer pink and cooked through, 4-5 minutes. Add marinara, bring to a boil, reduce heat and simmer 2-3 minutes. Remove pan from heat and cool slightly. Combine ricotta, spinach, parsley, egg whites, salt, and pepper in a large bowl. Coat the bottom of a 9 x 12 inch lasagna pan with ½ C sauce, arrange three lasagna noodles on the bottom of the pan. Spread ¾ C sauce evenly over noodles. Spoon 2/3 C ricotta-spinach mixture evenly on top of sauce. Repeat layers two more times. Cover top with three noodles and remaining ¾ C sauce. Sprinkle the mozzerella on top. Cover loosely with foil and bake for 45 minutes. Remove foil and bake 10-15 minutes, until cheese is bubbly. Cut into 9 squares and serve.

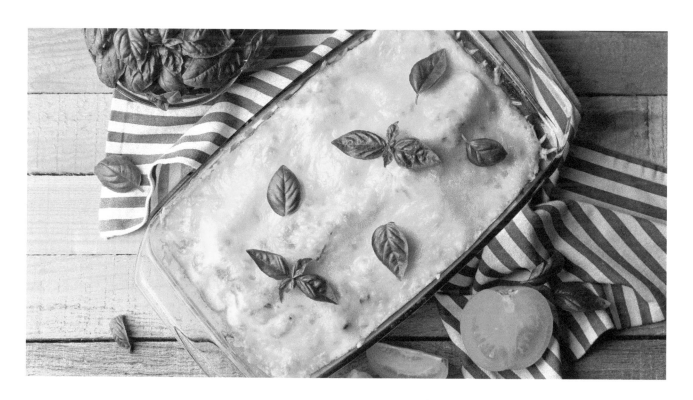

Rice bread w/ Sliced avocado
(Serves 1)

Ingredients:
Rice bread, 1 slice
Avocado (half)

Directions: Place one piece of rice bread in the toaster. Slice half of an avocado lengthwise and place on top of toast. Can also mash half an avocado onto the toast.

Garden Bean Soup
(See Page 25 Week 1 Sunday)

Kale Salad
(Serves 4)

Ingredients:
6 C kale, chopped
½ lemon
Pinch dried basil
Pinch sea salt
1 tbsp olive, camelina, flax or hemp seed oil
2 tbsp red onion, minced
2 tbsp green onion, chopped
1 small organic cucumber, thinly sliced
1 garlic clove, minced
¼ C chopped kalamata olives

Directions: Wash kale and cut into small strips. Steam for 5-7 min and transfer to bowl and add lemon, basil, salt and oil. Toss. Add the remaining ingredients and mix well.

Pumpkin Seed-Crusted Halibut
(Serves 2)

Ingredients:
½ tsp coriander
¼ C chopped raw pumpkin seeds
¼ C olive oil
1 lb halibut fillet, cut into two pieces
3 tbsp butter
1 lemon
1 tbsp chopped parsley

Directions: Preheat oven to 350 F. Add coriander to the pumpkin seeds and then chop the seeds in a food processor, being careful to avoid flour-like texture. Meanwhile, spread the olive oil over the bottom of a baking dish. Dredge the halibut through the olive oil so that all sides of the fish are lightly coated. With one hand, spoon the chopped pumpkin seeds onto all sides of the fish, while using the fingers of your other hand to pat the seeds onto the fish. Add 1.5 tbsp butter to the top of each piece of fish. Bake 10 minutes per inch of thickness. When done, squeeze lemon juice on each piece of fish and sprinkle with parsley.

7 Day Essential Diet Analysis

	Daily recommended intake	Total 7 day average:	Percentage 7 day average:
Calories	2000	2023.3	101.50%
From Carbohydrate	45-65% of diet	816.7	40.8% of diet
From Fat	20-35% of diet	820.4	41.0% of diet
From Protein	10-35% of diet	384.7	17.4% of diet
From Alcohol	0% of diet	~0	~0% of diet
Total Carbohydrate	300 g	214.6	71.50%
Dietary Fiber	21 g	43.9	209%
Starch	no RDA	14.2	–
Sugars	no RDA	64.3	–
Total Fat	65 g	95	146%
Saturated Fat	20 g	17.8	89%
Monounsaturated Fat	no RDA	43.3	–
Polyunsaturated Fat	no RDA	22	–
Trans Fat (g)	0	0.114	–
Total Omega-3 Fats	1100 mg	1720.2	156%
Total Omega-6 Fats	11000 mg	16888.4	154%

You are what you eat

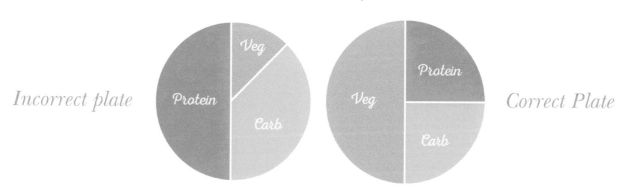

Incorrect plate — Protein, Veg, Carb

Correct Plate — Protein, Veg, Carb

Many diets are imbalanced between the amount of protein, vegetables and types of carbohydrates that people are consuming. If your plate looks like the one on the left above, shift your diet to include:
- 50% vegetables; 25% protein; 25% complex carbohydrates
- Consume healthy fats as parts of these categories by eating avocado, using healthy oils in salad dressings, and consuming fish and seafood.

A minimum of 20% of our daily recommended dietary intake needs to include healthy fats.

Below numbers are based on nutrients required for a 150lb (68kg) body weight.

	Daily recommended intake	Total: 7-day average Provided by The Essential Diet	Percentage: 7-day average Provided by The Essential Diet
Protein	0.8g/kg body weight	100.9	185%
Tryptophan (mg)	5 mg/kg body weight	988.6	290%
Threonine (mg)	20 mg/kg body weight	3141.3	231%
Isoleucine (mg)	19 mg/kg body weight	3685.9	285%
Leucine (mg)	42 mg/kg body weight	6103.7	213%
Lysine (mg)	38 mg/kg body weight	5494.6	212%
Methionine (mg)	19 mg/kg body weight	1760.1	136%
Cystine (mg)	19 mg/kg body weight	1050.6	81%
Phenylalanine (mg)	33 mg/kg body weight	3614.1	161%
Tyrosine (mg)	33 mg/kg body weight	2693.7	120%
Valine (mg)	24 mg/kg body weight	4204.3	257%
Arginine (mg)	not essential in adults	6263.4	-
Histidine (mg)	14 mg/kg body weight	2225	240%
Alanine (mg)	not essential	4195.4	-
Aspartic acid (mg)	not essential	8280.1	-
Glutamic acid (mg)	not essential	13989.4	-
Glycine (mg)	not essential	4159.9	-
Proline (mg)	not essential	3841.9	-
Serine (mg)	not essential	3694.3	-
Hydroxyproline (mg)	not essential	58.7	-
Vitamin A	2330 IU	26719.7	1146%
C	75 mg	168.1	224%
D	600IU	23.8	4%
E	22IU natural a-tocopherol	24.4	111%
K	90 mcg	925.3	1028%
Thiamin	1.1 mg	3.9	400%
Riboflavin	1.1 mg	3.9	400%
Niacin	14 mg	37.1	265%
Vitamin B6	1.3 mg	4.9	377%
Folate	400 mcg	627.7	157%
Vitamin B12	2.4 mg	3.9	163%
Pantothenic Acid	5 mg	5.1	105%
Choline	425 mg	277.1	65%
Betaine	no RDA	375	-
Calcium	1000 mg	674.3	67%
Iron	18 mg	22.3	123%
Magnesium	320 mg	623	195%
Phosphorus	700 mg	1574.6	225%
Potassium	4700 mg	3658.9	78%
Sodium	1500 mg	2395	160%
Zinc	8 mg	14.1	176%
Copper	0.9 mg	2.5	278%
Manganese	1.8 mg	7.22	401%
Selenium	55 mcg	74	134%
Fluoride	3 mg	32.1	1070%
Cholesterol	300 mg	198.9	66%
Phytosterols	no RDA	115.5	-
Caffeine	0 mg	0	-

Recipe references:

Morley, Carol. Delicious Detox
2010 - for: Green goddess; Blueberry buckwheat pancakes, Almond chicken, Asian asparagus, Flax baked chicken, Roasted beets and spinach salad, Berry-almond slam smoothie, Warm spicy sweet potato salad, Chickpea slaw, Fresh salad rolls and tangy almond dipping sauce.
Cookbook website: deliciousdetoxcookbook.com

Daniluk, Julie: Meals that Heal
Inflammation book, 2012 - for: Blueberry hemp smoothie; Crispy Kale Chips, Raw pad thai, Cranberry quiona salad, Grain-free berry muffins, Ginger butternut soup, Lentil dip, Arugula rainbow salad, Kale salad

Curried chicken salad
www.foodnetwork.com/recipes/tyler-florence/curried-chicken-salad-sandwich-with-almonds-and-raisins-recipe.html

Vegan mayo
www.thekitchn.com/how-to-make-easy-vegan-mayonnaise-227726

Salmon with balsamic glaze
www.foodnetwork.ca/recipe/grilled-salmon-with-balsamic-onion-glaze/9965/

Lentil vegetable soup
adapted from www.glutenfreeliving.com/recipes/soups-stews/vegan-lentil-soup/

Cornmeal carrot muffins
adapted from www.food.com/recipe/corn-carrot-muffins-190174

Ginger chicken stir fry
www.chatelaine.com/recipe/vegetables/ginger-chicken-stir-fry-with-greens/

Banana nut butter spread
www.blenderbabes.com/lifestyle-diet/dairy-free/banana-nut-butter-spread-recipe/

Soba noodle veggie pot
adapted from www.restlesspalate.com/asian-soba-noodles-purple-cabbage/

Three-bean vegetarian chili
www.myrecipes.com/recipe/three-bean-vegetarian-chili

Apple and Hazelnut muesli
www.theguardian.com/lifeandstyle/wordofmouth/2014/oct/23/how-to-make-perfect-bircher-muesli-recipe

No-noodle zucchini lasagna
www.allrecipes.com/recipe/172958/no-noodle-zucchini-lasagna/

Crispy breakfast bars
www.vegetariantimes.com/recipe/crispy-breakfast-bars/

Shrimp in thai green curry
www.thaikitchen.com/Recipes/Seafood/Green-Curry-Shrimp

Breakfast sausage
adapted from www.healthylivinghowto.com/1/post/2012/07/say-goodbye-to-jimmy-dean.html

Wonderful whatever salad
from book AARP The Inflammation Syndrome: Your Nutrition Plan for Great Health, Weight Loss, and Pain-Free Living by Jack Challem

Vegetarian Chili with avocado salsa
from myrecipes.com: www.myrecipes.com/recipe/quick-vegetarian-chili-with-avocado-salsa

Sesame seed crusted salmon burgers
from Health magazine www.health.com/health/recipe/0,,1000000199042,00.html

Edamame and bean salad with shrimp and fresh salsa
from myrecipes.com: www.myrecipes.com/recipe/edamame-bean-salad-with-shrimp-fresh-salsa

Spaghetti squash and black bean tacos
from The Smitten Kitchen cookbook, adjusted here www.blueberriesandbasil.wordpress.com/2015/09/24/smitten-kitchens-spaghetti-squash-tacos-with-black-beans-and-queso-fresco/

Stewed kale and lentils
www.canadianliving.com/food/quick-and-easy/recipe/stewed-kale-and-lentils

Warm oat and apple bowl
from the GL Cookbook and Diet Plan, by Nigel Denby, 2007 www.amazon.com/Cookbook-Diet-Plan-Weight-Loss-Delicious/dp/1569756112

Garden Bean soup
adapted from www.myrecipes.com/recipe/curried-lentil-chickpea-stew

Pumpkin-seed crusted Halibut
www.epicurious.com/recipes/food/views/grilled-halibut-with-coriander-pepita-butter-353330

Index